Allergies

S0-FLR-090

By Judy Monroe

Consultant:
Michael Wein, MD
Fellow, American College of Allergy, Asthma, Immunology
Chief of Allergy, Indian River Memorial Hospital
Vero Beach, Florida

Perspectives on Disease and Illness

LifeMatters
an imprint of Capstone Press
Mankato, Minnesota

LifeMatters Books are published by Capstone Press
PO Box 669 • 151 Good Counsel Drive • Mankato, Minnesota 56002
http://www.capstone-press.com

©2001 Capstone Press. All rights reserved. No part of this book may be reproduced or transmitted in any form or by any means without written permission from the publisher. The publisher takes no responsibility for the use of any of the materials or methods described in this book nor for the products thereof.

Printed in the United States of America

Library of Congress Cataloging-in-Publication Data
Monroe, Judy.
     Allergies / by Judy Monroe.
          p.   cm. — (Perspectives on disease and illness)
     Includes bibliographical references and index.
     ISBN 0-7368-0752-7
     1. Allergy—Juvenile literature. [1. Allergy.] I. Title. II. Series.
     RC585 .M66 2001
     616.97—dc21   00-009680
                                                                                             CIP

     Summary: Describes allergies, including hay fever and skin, food, and other allergies. Describes methods doctors use to diagnose, treat, and control allergies. Includes ways to handle an allergy attack.

Staff Credits
Charles Pederson, editor; Adam Lazar, designer; Kim Danger, photo researcher
Cover production by Anne Schafer
Interior production by Stacey Field

Photo Credits
Cover: ©DigitalVision, left; ©Artville/Simiji, middle; ©DigitalVision, right; StockMarket/©Chris Jones, bottom
Photo Agora/©Jeff J. Daly, 16; ©Richard Martin, 40
Photo Network/©Carol Christensen, 15
Photri, 59
Unicorn/©Ron P. Jaffe, 7; ©Rod Furgason, 8; ©Aneal E. Vohra, 21; ©Chris Boylan, 33; ©Eric R. Berndt, 36; ©Jeff Greenberg, 45, 50; ©Ted Rose, 48
Visuals Unlimited/©Jeff Greenberg, 11; ©Robert Clay, 20; ©Ken Greer, 25; ©M & D Long, 27; ©Bernd Wittich, 28; ©William J. Weber, 35; ©WIHC, 42; ©John Trager, 57

A 0 9 8 7 6 5 4 3 2 1

Table of Contents

1	What Are Allergies?	4
2	Seasonal Hay Fever	12
3	Skin and Food Allergies	22
4	Other Types of Allergies	30
5	Diagnosing Allergies	38
6	Controlling Allergies	46
7	Handling an Allergy Attack	54
	Glossary	60
	For More Information	61
	Useful Addresses and Internet Sites	62
	Index	63

Chapter Overview

Having an allergy means being sensitive to certain substances that most people don't react to. Many things people breathe, eat, touch, or take into their body can cause an allergy.

Allergy is a big cause of poor health in children. Allergies affect millions of people worldwide. In North America, allergies affect about one in five people. Allergies can vary from mild to severe or even deadly.

During an allergic reaction, many symptoms may occur. The eyes may water and the nose run. The mouth and throat might itch. Breathing may be difficult, and some people wheeze and sneeze. Sometimes a rash, itchy red bumps, or a stomachache occurs.

Substances that cause an allergic reaction are called allergens or allergy triggers. Common allergy triggers include pollen, mold, insects, and animals.

Allergies often run in families but can affect people of all races and ages.

Chapter 1

What Are Allergies?

"We always get the same pizza. Let's try a different one," said Tyler. His friends agreed and ordered a shrimp pizza. Tyler and his friends ate it up. Then they went to a nearby video arcade.

Tyler, Age 15

Tyler was playing when he said, "My face feels itchy."

Lee frowned. "You sound funny. Your lips are swollen and your eyes are red. I don't think you should scratch those red spots on your face. What's wrong with you, Tyler?"

Tyler had an allergic reaction. His body reacted in unusual ways to shrimp. People with allergies can be sensitive to many different foods, plants, and animals. People can be allergic to many things they breathe, eat, touch, or take into the body. However, most things are unlikely to cause an allergy.

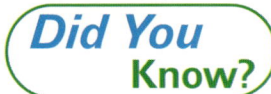

Did You Know?

The word *allergy* comes from two Greek words. *Allos* means "other" and *ergon* means "work." An allergy changes how the body works or reacts to certain substances. The word *allergy* was first used in English in 1906.

An allergy can be chronic, or long lasting. An allergy even may last a lifetime. Some allergies disappear as children and teens grow older. Allergies can reappear later in life, and new allergies can develop at any time.

Allergies affect millions of people worldwide. In North America, one out of five people has an allergy. That adds up to about 50 million people in the United States. About 10 to 15 percent of all children in North America have one or more allergies. Some people experience seasonal allergies such as hay fever. Others may have year-round allergies.

Allergies are a major cause of ill health in children. Sometimes allergies can be severe. In rare instances, an allergic reaction can be deadly. If not treated, allergies can reduce a person's ability to do everyday activities. For example, teens with asthma may not be able to play sports. Asthma is a lung disorder. People with asthma sometimes find it difficult to breathe during an asthma attack. Untreated allergies also can result in other chronic problems such as skin disorders.

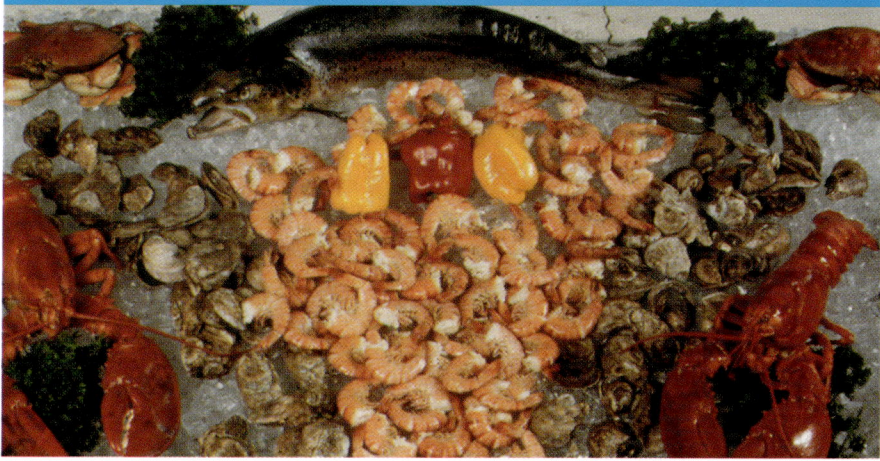

Seafood and shellfish are common allergy triggers.

An Immune System Disorder

To understand allergies, it's helpful to know about the immune system, which protects the body from illness and disease. The immune system includes cells contained in glands, the skin, the stomach, and the blood. Normally, the immune system successfully fights pathogens. These are things that can make people sick, such as bacteria and viruses.

The immune system does a good job most of the time. Special white blood cells in the immune system produce large molecules called antibodies to fight off harmful invaders. Each antibody fights one particular substance. The immune system produces the correct antibodies each time a harmful substance enters the body.

Sometimes, however, the immune system gets mixed up. It may mistakenly attack harmless substances such as shrimp or pollen. Then the special white blood cells produce antibodies against these things. The antibodies cause the lining in the eyes and nose to release chemicals. One is called histamine. In turn, histamine causes an allergic reaction complete with miserable symptoms.

During an allergic reaction, your nose may be runny.

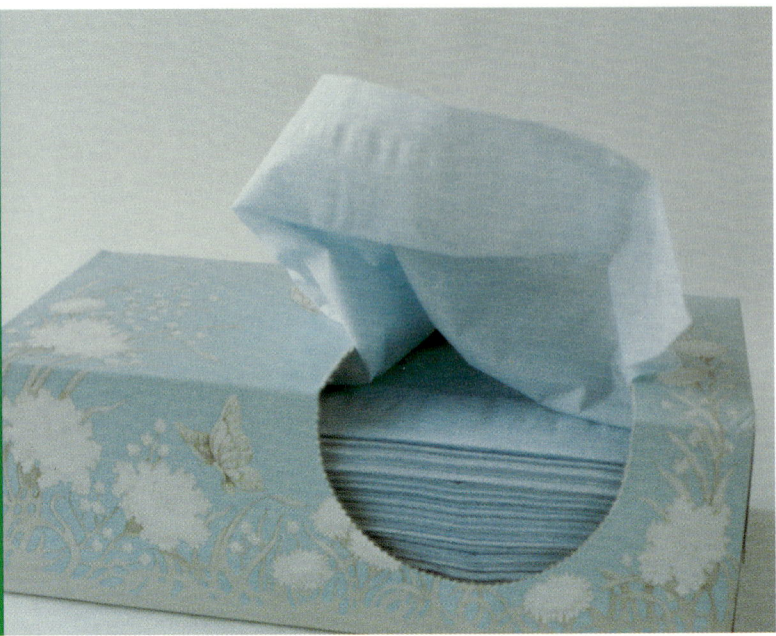

During an allergic reaction, many things can happen. The eyes may water or turn red, and the nose might run. The mouth and throat could itch. Breathing may be more difficult, and some people wheeze and sneeze. Sometimes, a rash, a stomachache, or itchy red bumps called hives appear. All this usually happens minutes after the allergy-causing substance touches or enters the body. Chapter 5 describes how symptoms help to diagnose allergies, or figure out what they are.

Allergy Triggers

Hundreds of substances can make people with allergies feel uncomfortable or sick. These substances are called allergens. They sometimes are called allergy triggers because they stimulate an allergic reaction. Allergy triggers vary from person to person. Many foods, plants, or animals are or contain allergens. The chart shows many common allergy triggers.

Myth: Allergies don't affect a person's day-to-day life.

Fact: Allergies affect many people. The United States loses 3.5 million workdays yearly from allergies. This missed time adds up to $639 million lost each year. Children and teens lose about 2 million days of school every year. Over 8 million people see doctors every year for relief from hay fever.

Myth vs. Fact

Possible Allergy Triggers

Pollen, or dustlike plant substance that is needed to produce new plants	Insulin, or a substance that the body produces to help use blood sugar
Dust mites, or tiny spiderlike creatures	Foods
Animal saliva, skin, or urine	Drugs in liquid or pill form
Mold	Dyes
Insect parts and droppings	Latex rubber
Vaccines, or preparations of dead bacteria to help fight disease	Metals
	Cosmetic ingredients in makeup, cologne, perfume, nail polish
Insect stings	Weeds, grass, trees

What Are Allergies?

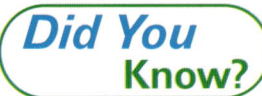

Did You Know? Allergies and asthma often go together. At least 80 percent of children and half of adults with asthma have one or more allergies.

The Chang Family

The entire Chang family seems to be allergic to something. Mrs. Chang loves horses, but she wheezes and can't catch her breath when she's around them. Pearl, age 16, gets hay fever every summer. She sneezes a lot, and her eyes water and itch. She developed hay fever 10 years ago and can't eat apples and cherries because of it. Her mouth feels tingly when she does. Sing, the baby, is allergic to cow's milk, so Mrs. Chang gives her soy milk instead.

Who Gets Allergies?

Allergies tend to run in families, as they seem to in the Chang family. Children are more likely to develop allergies if their parents have allergies. A child has a 25 percent chance of developing allergies if one parent is allergic. That rate can more than double if both parents are allergic to something. On the other hand, just because someone in the family has an allergy doesn't mean others will have one.

Clay, Age 13, and Tom, Age 15

Clay and Tom are brothers who look alike. They both like to hike, camp, and fish. They eat the same foods, live in the same house, and go to the same school. However, their health histories are different. Clay has chronic allergies to various things such as pollen, molds, house dust, and milk. Tom has no allergies.

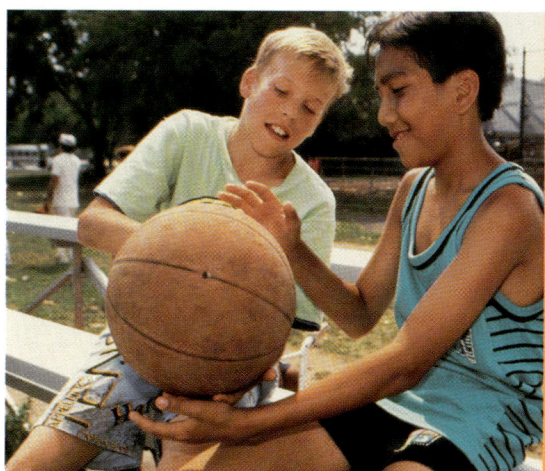

Allergies can affect people of all ages and races.

Some people might not inherit an allergy itself but might inherit a tendency to get one. They only need something to trigger it. Specific allergy triggers and symptoms of allergies vary from person to person. Most people have only one or two allergies. Others may have more. An allergy isn't contagious. It can't pass from person to person like a cold or the flu.

Allergies affect people of all races and ages. Children with allergies can have more serious reactions than adults with allergies. Sometimes allergies lessen as infants and children get older. This is because the immune system matures and can better handle allergies.

Points to Consider

Name one fact you learned about allergies after reading this chapter. Were you surprised by this information? Why or why not?

Do you or does anyone you know have an allergy? What is an allergic reaction like for you or this person?

What do you think would happen if your immune system stopped working?

Chapter Overview

Hay fever is often seasonal and occurs in warm weather months. Hay fever affects about one-fifth of all North Americans.

Pollen is the most common trigger for hay fever. The main allergen is pollen from certain trees, grasses, and weeds.

Another common hay fever trigger is mold, which grows best in damp places. People can be allergic to one or more types of mold.

People can control hay fever.

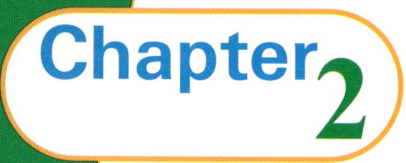

Seasonal Hay Fever

Most people look forward to being outside in the warm weather. However, some people dread the warmth. They know it's the prime time of year for pollen and molds, which cause hay fever. People don't like to feel miserable because of hay fever. Let's take a look at it.

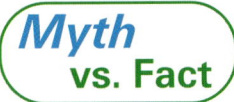

Myth: Hay fever is a fever in people who are allergic to hay.

Fact: Hay fever has nothing to do with hay and never causes a fever.

> Josh has hay fever. He feels sick every spring and summer and can't stay outdoors for more than a few minutes. He explains, "I feel really bad. My nose and head get all stuffed up. My eyes keep watering. The back of my throat itches. Sometimes I'll sneeze 20 times in a row and then get a bad headache."
>
> **Josh, Age 17**

What Is Hay Fever?

Worldwide, spring begins the season for the most common allergy, allergic rhinitis. A more common name for allergic rhinitis is hay fever. Weeds and new growth on trees trigger hay fever.

People with hay fever react to outdoor allergens such as pollen or mold. These are in the air at certain times, and the wind blows them around. Some particles land on cells in the nose, sinus cavities in the head, airways, and eyes. In someone with hay fever, the cells release histamine and other chemical substances. These substances irritate the lining of the nose, cavities inside the head, eyelids, and eyes. Body tissue in these areas can turn red and swell up. These symptoms can make people feel miserable.

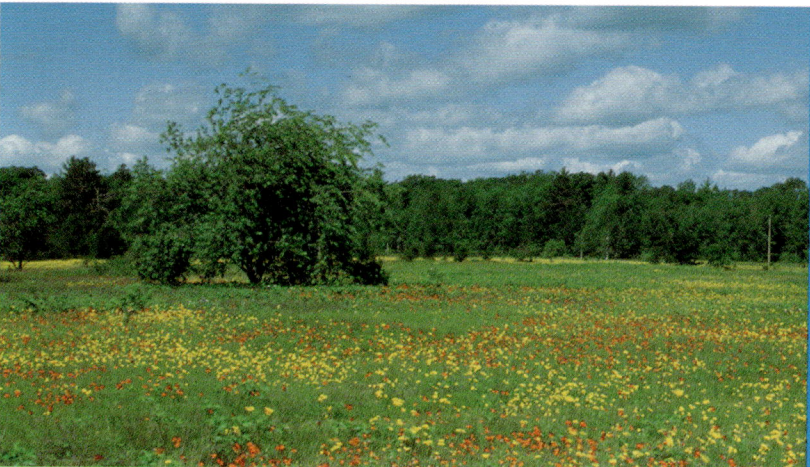

Flower pollen can cause allergies.

Some people's hay fever symptoms are mild. Other people feel terrible all the time. Hay fever can cause a sore throat and headache. Symptoms may become so severe that people sleep poorly or have difficulty breathing. They may begin to feel tired and irritable.

Who Gets Hay Fever?

Hay fever affects 18 to 20 percent of North Americans. About 35 million people in the United States alone have hay fever. This number is on the increase, though experts aren't sure why.

Hay fever can start at any age, and both males and females can develop it. It often first appears in people between ages 12 and 16. For some teens, hay fever becomes chronic. Other people find that it lessens or even disappears later in life. Some people first develop hay fever as an adult.

Pollen Triggers for Hay Fever

The most common hay fever trigger is ragweed pollen. Every plant that makes seeds produces pollen. These tiny grains are too small to be seen with the naked eye, but they are all around us.

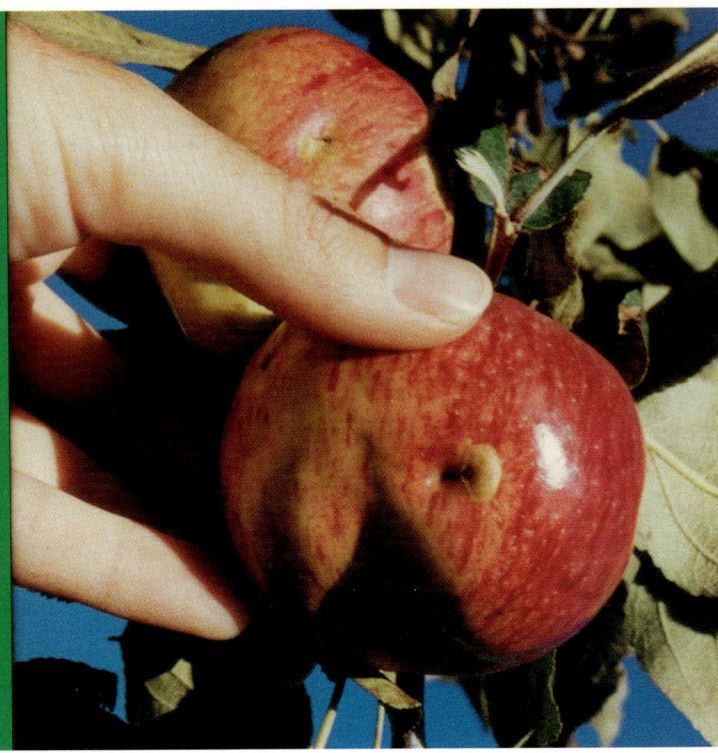

People with allergies to birch tree pollen sometimes react to apples, cherries, peaches, pears, or carrots.

Many plants produce large amounts of pollen. Just one flowering bush may produce hundreds of millions of pollen particles. The wind carries the lightest pollens that cause the most allergies. Insects, birds, and bats also spread pollen.

Pollens that cause allergies vary by season. Tree pollen is the main allergen in the spring. In the summer, grass pollen often triggers hay fever. Weed pollen hits in the fall. People can be allergic to one pollen or several. For example, some people may be allergic to either ragweed or grass pollen. Other people may be allergic to both.

Some plants produce more pollen than others and are most likely to cause hay fever. The chart shows several common pollen allergens.

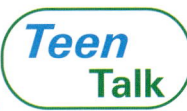

"My parents want to move to Arizona. The warm, dry air is supposed to help Dad's hay fever. I asked the school nurse about this, and she said that's not true. Moving to warm, dry areas may relieve hay fever for a few months. But new allergies to local plants can develop. She said no part of North America is free of plants that cause hay fever."—Jerry, age 14

Examples of Pollen Types

Tree

Ash	Oak
Beech	Pecan
Birch	Poplar
Elm	Sycamore
Hickory	Western red cedar
Maple	

Grass

Bermuda	Orchard
Johnson	Red top
June	Rye
Kentucky blue	Sweet vernal
Meadow fescue	Timothy

Weed

English plantain	Sagebrush
Lamb's quarters	Sheep sorrel
Ragweed	Tumbleweed (Russian thistle)
Red root pigweed	

Seasonal Hay Fever

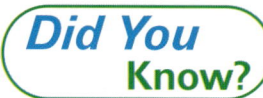 You don't need to be nearby for a plant's pollen to affect you. The wind can carry pollen for hundreds of miles.

Mold

Along with pollen, mold is another common hay fever trigger. Molds are tiny living creatures that grow outdoors and indoors. Molds grow best in damp places. Thousands of types of molds exist, but only a few dozen cause most allergies. People can be allergic to one or more types.

The outdoor mold season often starts in the spring and ends in the fall. In North America, the worst months are usually from July to late fall. In warm areas, mold allergies can last all year.

Indoors, mold can grow anywhere with enough moisture to keep it alive. A home that feels damp or has a musty smell often has a lot of mold. Bathrooms, kitchens, and basements are favorite places for molds. So are refrigerators, garbage containers, carpets, pillows, and mattresses.

Smoke, insect sprays, and tar fumes aren't allergens but can worsen hay fever symptoms.

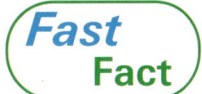

Outdoors, molds can grow in many places. They can form on leaf piles, soil, woodpiles, and other moist surfaces. Other common areas are:

Freshly mowed grass
Poorly drained areas
Haystacks and grain bins
Garbage cans
Camping equipment
Lawnmowers
Golf bags
Vehicles—under floor mats and in the air conditioning system

The wind blows tiny pieces of mold around. They may enter homes from outside through open doors and windows. People can have an allergic reaction when they breathe in the pieces or get them in the eyes.

Coping With Hay Fever Triggers

Various ways exist to control hay fever. Some people stay indoors early in the morning or on warm, dry, windy days. These are times when pollen counts are at their highest. People may do outdoor activities such as yard work in the afternoon or evening. They may avoid yard work where mold growth is heavy or ask someone else to do the work for them. Wearing a dust mask helps keep mold and pollen out of the mouth and nose.

Pollen can cling to clothing that's dried outdoors.

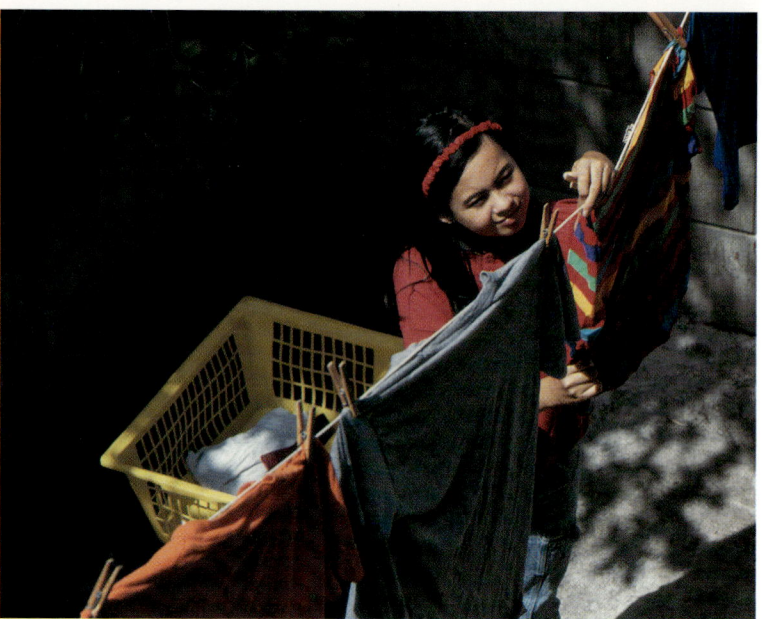

Here are some ways to reduce indoor pollen:

> Shower after being outdoors.
>
> Wash clothes that were worn outside, then dry them in a dryer. Clothes dried outdoors can catch and hold pollen.
>
> Keep house and car windows and doors closed.
>
> Run the air conditioner or turn on the furnace fan. This helps filter out pollen. Clean or change air conditioner filters once a month.

To deal with mold allergy, reduce mold levels. Outside, keep the grass short, shrubs trimmed, and the yard clean. This lets in sunlight and dries out the area. Get rid of standing water in the yard. Mold has a hard time growing on moving water or in dry areas. Remove compost heaps or bins. Inside, use a dehumidifier to help keep the basement or other damp rooms dry. Empty the water regularly to prevent mold growth in the machine. The best relative humidity, or moisture in the air, is 50 percent or less.

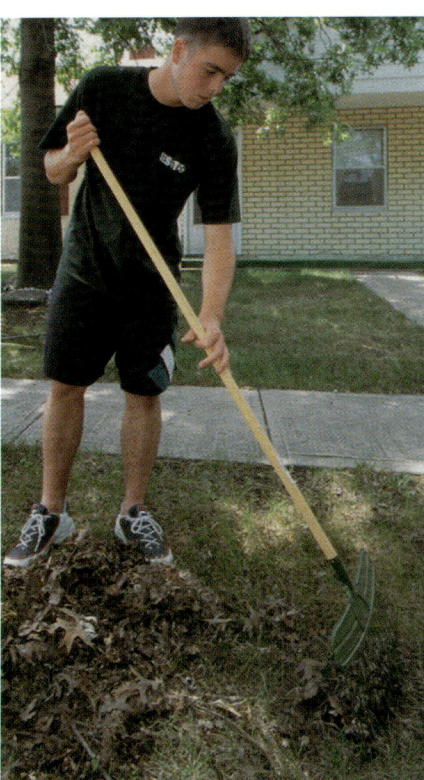

Keeping your yard clean is a good way to reduce pollen and mold in the yard.

Dave, Age 15

Dave lived in northern Minnesota. Like his dad, he wanted to be a carpenter. Unlike his dad, he sneezed all the time when he worked outdoors. The doctor said that Dave had a mold allergy. Carpenters often work in places with high levels of mold. The doctor said that Dave might want to think about other career choices.

Points to Consider

Do you know anyone who could have hay fever? What would you say to the person?

Write down some ways you could reduce mold or pollen indoors or outdoors where you live.

People in warm areas have longer periods of hay fever than people in colder areas. Why do you think that's true?

Chapter Overview

People with a skin allergy react to an allergen that touches the skin. An itchy rash is the most common reaction.

Many different substances can cause skin allergies. Common allergens include poison ivy, poison oak, and poison sumac. Another common skin allergy is allergic eczema.

Food allergies are not common. Most food allergies involve protein in foods such as nuts, peanuts, shellfish, milk, wheat, or soy. Typical symptoms are similar to other allergy symptoms.

The best way to control skin or food allergies is to avoid the allergen. Reading food labels and consulting an allergist or dietitian also can help you avoid food allergies.

Chapter 3

Skin and Food Allergies

Like most allergies, skin allergies are common and on the increase. They're the most common skin condition in children younger than 11 years old. Food allergies are less common, although almost 25 percent of people think they're allergic to something. The fact is, in North America, only 3 percent of children and 1 percent of adults have a food allergy.

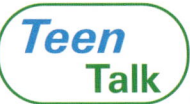

"My eyelids were red, itchy, swollen, and sore. Dad said it was my nail polish. I didn't believe him, so I went to a doctor. What do you know? Dad was right! The doctor told me I really was allergic to some of the chemicals in the polish. I threw it away, and in a few days, my eyelids looked and felt okay."
—Hannah, age 17

Teshia, Age 18

Teshia was a senior in high school. She loved computers and helped out in the family business. One weekend, Teshia worked with her mom to set up a new computer billing system. She printed off all the old and new bills. For this big job, she used up several boxes of new printer paper. By Sunday night, Teshia's hands, arms, and face were covered with a rash. Her family discovered later that Teshia had a skin allergy to a chemical in the paper.

What Are Skin Allergies?

Skin allergies occur when some people get an allergic reaction when they touch certain substances. Within 12 to 48 hours after touching an allergen, these people usually develop an itchy rash. It can appear on any part of the skin. It most often occurs on the hands and face, or in areas where the skin is thin. The skin on the eyelids and neck are other likely places for a rash.

Allergy rashes are often dry and scaly. They may burn and become red and irritated. Blisters can appear. The rash may last from a few days to weeks. Sometimes bacteria get into the area, and a serious infection develops.

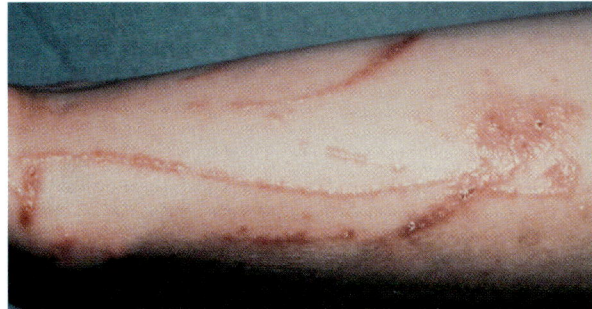

Poison ivy caused this person's allergic rash.

About 2,800 different substances are known to cause skin allergies. There may be others that aren't yet known. Plants are the most common allergens. For example, poison ivy, oak, and sumac cause an allergic reaction in about 70 percent of the U.S. population. Hair dye is another common cause of allergies.

Less common allergens include everyday things such as cement, perfume, flour, or detergent. Other allergens are nickel, chrome, and mercury, which are metals. Nickel is often used in jewelry, including up to 14-carat gold. Nickel can be found in keys, zippers, snaps, and hooks. More things with nickel are needles, scissors, doorknobs, and coins.

Allergic Eczema

Another common skin allergy is allergic eczema. This chronic condition causes itchy, scaly skin rashes. The itching often begins before the rash develops. Areas of eczema can become infected with bacteria. If this happens, severe skin infections can result.

Eczema occurs more often in children than in adults. In North Americans, it often appears in people before age 2. However, eczema can affect people of any age. As many as 2 percent of people in the United States have eczema. It tends to run in families. Doctors don't know what causes eczema, and it may disappear as children and teens get older.

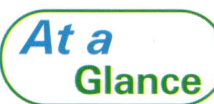

Latex can cause skin allergies in some people. Latex comes from the milky liquid from the rubber tree. Many products contain latex, such as some rubber gloves, condoms, erasers, balloons, bandages, and tires. About 1 percent of people in the United States have this allergy. Health care workers have a greater chance of developing a latex allergy than other people do.

Coping With Skin Allergies

The best way to deal with a skin allergy is to avoid the allergen. If that's impossible, other steps can head off skin allergies. Wash skin, clothing, and items that come into contact with allergens. Use soap and warm water and rinse well. Poison ivy can stay on clothes and tools for months. Unless washed away, it can cause a reaction months later if touched.

Don't scratch an allergy rash. Scratching can spread the allergen to other parts of the skin. Put ice packs on the rash to soothe the itching. Wear gloves when using possible allergens. Use unscented products, including paper products. Perfume and other scents sometimes cause allergies in people.

What Are Food Allergies?

Many people think they have a food allergy. They may have an intolerance to some foods, but actual food allergies are rare. Real food allergies cause changes in the immune system. The body makes antibodies when a person eats certain foods. The antibodies trigger the release of histamine and other chemicals. In turn, histamine causes many symptoms of food allergies.

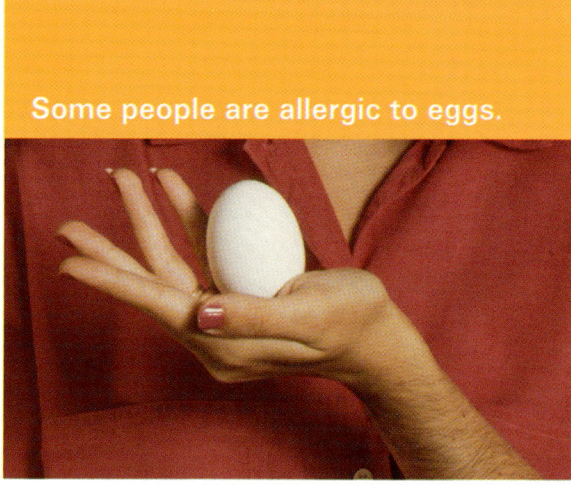
Some people are allergic to eggs.

The symptoms of a food allergy vary. Along with typical allergy symptoms, a person may have swollen lips, tongue, hands, or face, and stomach pain or diarrhea. This occurs when normally solid waste becomes loose and runny. Some people have breathing problems, feel dizzy or sick, or even faint. Food allergy reactions occur in seconds, minutes, or hours. In uncommon cases, food allergies can be deadly.

Most food allergies involve protein found in certain foods. For adults, the top four allergens are nuts, peanuts, shellfish, and fish. Other allergens include milk, soy, or wheat. Eggs, milk, and peanuts are the most common food allergens for children.

Who Gets Food Allergies?

Nonfood allergies are more common than food allergies. But anyone can develop a food allergy at any age. Most food allergies occur among people with a family history of allergies.

Children are more likely to have food allergies than adults are. Many children outgrow their food allergies when they become teens. They're more likely to outgrow allergies to milk and soy than to other foods. Adults seldom lose their food allergies.

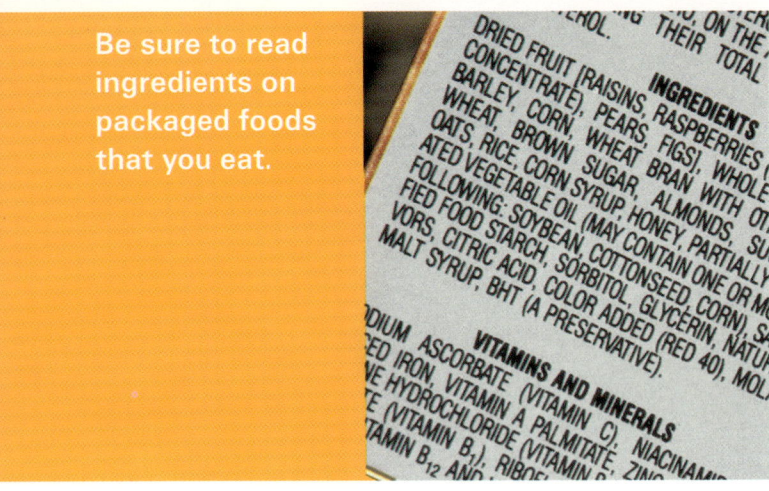

Be sure to read ingredients on packaged foods that you eat.

Coping With Food Allergies

The best way to deal with a food allergy is to avoid the problem food. That can be hard to do at times. One way is to read food labels. Watch out, though. The food may be listed under a different name. If you're unsure, call the company and ask what their product contains. Many food companies have toll-free phone numbers.

Food companies sometimes change their products. They may add or remove ingredients. Be sure to check labels every time you buy a food product.

> **Estela, Age 15**
>
> Estela reads all labels on prepared foods she eats. Any food that contains wheat products will make her sick. "This allergy is no fun. I can't eat pizza. I can't have a sandwich or pancakes. I can't eat snacks such as crackers or cookies. Most sauces are off-limits for me. Most use wheat to thicken the sauce. It's amazing how many foods contain some type of wheat. Even soy sauce. I've gotten good at reading food labels."

For people with food allergies, eating out can be tricky. Ask the server or chef about the foods on the menu. If in doubt, don't eat the food. Or pack a tasty meal to eat away from home.

At a Glance

Here are food label ingredients to watch for if you're allergic to milk, eggs, or wheat:

Milk: Casein, whey, lactalbumin, lactose, cream, curds

Eggs: Albumin, mayonnaise, ovalbumin

Wheat: Flour, gluten, food starch, vegetable starch, bran, farina

---

At home, clean cutting boards or counters touched by foods that trigger an allergy. Wash with soap and hot water. Use clean plates, forks, spoons, and knives.

People with food allergies can get help from allergists or dietitians. These experts can teach people which foods to avoid. They also can give ideas for substitute foods.

Points to Consider

Do you know what poison oak, ivy, and sumac look like? How could you find this information?

How could you help someone with a skin or food allergy?

Why do you think so many people believe they have a food allergy? What could cause their discomfort when they eat some foods?

Why do you think children outgrow some food allergies?

What would you say if someone said, "Food allergies aren't serious"?

Chapter Overview

Dust allergies are common in the United States. Dust mites are the most common allergy trigger in dust.

Animal allergens are the saliva, dander, or urine of an animal. People can have an allergy to one or more animals.

Cockroaches can trigger allergy attacks. These pests live in many places including homes. They need water and like moist areas with plenty of food.

A drug allergy is a reaction to a drug. Drug allergies aren't as common as nonallergic drug reactions.

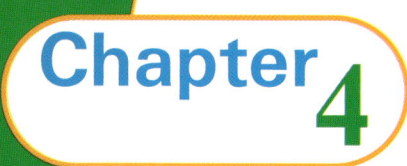

Chapter 4

Other Types of Allergies

Besides pollen, mold, skin, and food allergies, other types of allergies occur. At the top of the list are allergies to dust and dust mites, pets, cockroaches, and drugs.

Dust and Dust Mites

Indoor dust can cause allergic reactions in some people. It's a difficult allergy to deal with because dust is almost everywhere. About 10 to 15 percent of people in the United States have a dust allergy. It often lasts throughout the year. This allergy's symptoms are typical of those of pollen or mold allergies.

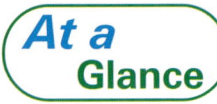

At a Glance

Dust mites aren't insects but are part of the spider family. Dust mites are too small to be seen with the naked eye. Over 200 million dust mites can live in one bed! Dust mites have no eyes or wings and can't drink. Instead, they get water from the air through special leg parts. Other than causing allergies, dust mites are harmless.

House dust is made up of small bits of plant and animal material. Dust mites are the most common allergen in dust in the home. These tiny creatures eat skin that people and other animals shed. The droppings and dead bodies of dust mites cause allergic reactions.

Dust mites need moisture to live. They thrive in warm, humid places and are found in most homes. Dust mites like fabrics such as carpets, curtains, and drapes. Other favorite places for dust mites are mattresses, pillows, and blankets. All of these contain many dead skin flakes.

Coping With Dust and Dust Mites

There are three main ways to control dust mites. First, keep indoor humidity below 50 percent. An air conditioner can help lower humidity.

Second, reduce the amount of house dust. Clean often. Use a damp cloth or mop to pick up dust.

Page 32   Allergies

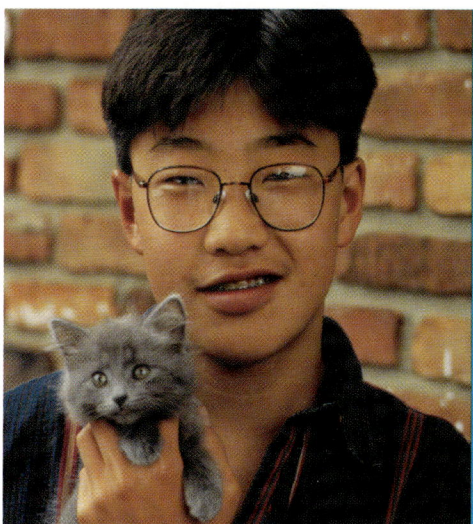

Pets can cause allergies. For example, cat dander or saliva can be allergens.

Third, get rid of favorite dust mite places. Replace curtains and drapes with plastic shades or blinds. Remove rugs and carpeting if possible. Put clothing into drawers or closets so it doesn't get dusty. Cover beds and pillows with allergy-proof covers. These are available at many stores. Some new beds and pillows have special coatings that make them free from allergens.

> **Lily, Age 14**
>
> Lily likes dogs but can't have one because of a severe allergy. On vacation, Lily and her family were going to stay in a motel. They pulled in by early afternoon. Soon, Lily and her family unpacked and put away their clothes. After 20 minutes, Lily began to sneeze and rub her eyes. "This feels like my dog allergy," she said. "Someone must have had a dog here."

Pets

Lily was right. People can keep dogs in some hotel and motel rooms. A dog had been in Lily's room for a week and had just left that morning. Lily's parents had forgotten to request a no-pet room. The room was clean, but the cleaner couldn't pick up all the dog allergens.

Other Types of Allergies

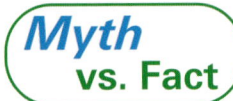

Myth: Removing a pet will make the allergen disappear right away.

Fact: Pet allergens won't disappear immediately. Research shows that cat allergens remain in a room up to six months after the cat is gone.

Animal allergies are an immune system response to an allergen in an animal's saliva, dander, or urine. Dander is tiny flakes of skin. People can be allergic to one or more kinds of pets. Cats and dogs are the most common. Other allergies are to horses, rabbits, hamsters, mice, rats, or birds. People with a pet allergy often have many symptoms that are like pollen or mold allergies. If the pet is indoors, these symptoms will exist all the time.

Animal allergies are increasing in North America as more and more people have pets. Between 5 and 10 percent of the U.S. population is allergic to mammals such as cats and dogs.

Coping With a Pet Allergy

Someone with a severe allergy to an animal may not be able to keep a pet. Getting rid of a family pet can be difficult for everyone in the family. Sometimes people will decide not to part with their pets. Instead, they look for ways to keep their pets and control their allergy.

Here are some things that can help:

- Wash the pet every week.
- Change bedsheets regularly and keep blankets and pillows clean.
- Keep the house free of dust.
- Run the air conditioner and keep the air filter clean. High efficiency particle arresting (HEPA) filters work best.

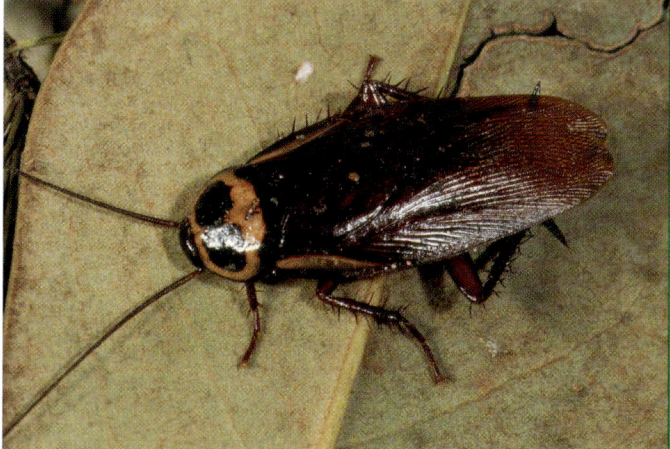

Call a pest-control professional to get rid of cockroaches if they're in your home.

Cockroaches

Cockroaches are common insects with long legs and a flat, hard body. Most cockroaches live outdoors. Others live in homes, offices, and restaurants. They need water and like moist areas with plenty of food.

Cockroach bodies and droppings can trigger allergy attacks. This material collects as house dust and is hard to remove. Cockroaches trigger allergy attacks most often in crowded living conditions.

A trained pest-control person can get rid of cockroaches once they enter a home. Some stores sell roach traps and sprays. Following are nonpoisonous ways to keep cockroaches out of a home:

> Seal areas where cockroaches can enter. This includes wall and floor cracks or gaps, drains, windows, and outside doors.
>
> Clean often, especially the kitchen. Wash dirty dishes right away. Put food into well-sealed containers. Remove any food bits under stoves, refrigerators, and toasters. Wipe off the stove, counters, and kitchen table and keep the floor clean.
>
> Take all garbage outside as soon as possible.

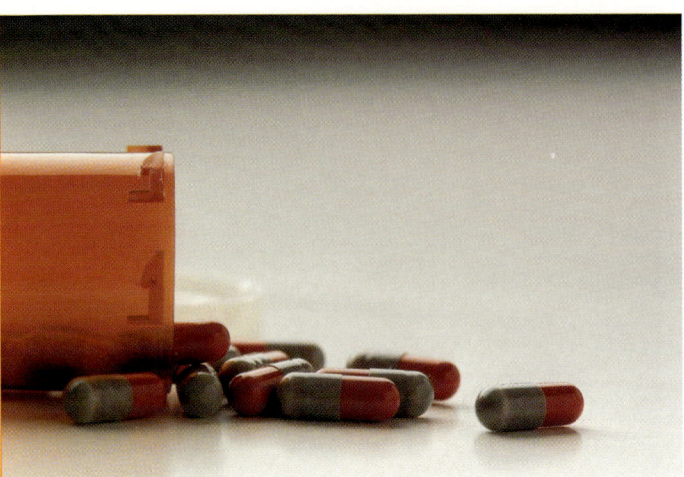

Pills are less common sources of allergies than medicines given by shot.

Drugs

A drug allergy occurs as the body absorbs and uses a drug. Drug allergies do occur, but less often than other drug side effects. The immune system doesn't trigger these unwanted and unpleasant symptoms.

Drug allergy symptoms include most typical ones for other allergies. Other symptoms include abdominal pain, diarrhea, and throwing up.

Rarely, drug allergy symptoms can be serious enough to kill a person. Symptoms often occur within minutes to hours after taking the drug. Other times, the allergy shows up after continued use. Some drugs such as penicillin are more likely than others to cause allergic reactions. Penicillin is a medicine used to treat several diseases and infections. Drugs taken as pills are less likely to cause serious allergies than drugs taken as shots.

Drug allergies can develop at any age. They may disappear over time. People allergic to one drug also may react to similar ones. The best way to cope with a drug allergy is to avoid the drug. You often can find other ways to treat a health problem than with drugs.

Laurel had a small red rash on her arm. She wanted to wear a sleeveless top to her friend's house the next day. Laurel's dad bought some lotion at the drugstore. It was supposed to get rid of the rash. At first, it seemed to help. Then the rash got worse. It turned bright red and itched a lot. Laurel went to the doctor, who said, "Your rash would have gone away on its own. The medicine you've been using made it worse. You're allergic to an ingredient in it."

Laurel, Age 15

Points to Consider

Bedrooms often have high levels of dust mites. What might be some reasons for this?

Someone with dust or pet allergies should avoid cleaning with a broom. Why do you think that's true?

Why can regularly bathing a pet help someone with an animal allergy?

How could you help friends who have to give up their pets because of allergies?

Chapter Overview

It's important to diagnose an allergy. Allergies can be serious for people with severe reactions.

The main symptoms of an allergy are sneezing, hives, rashes, and itchy eyes, nose, mouth, or skin.

Doctors diagnose allergies based on a person's symptoms, medical history, and skin tests. Skin tests are the most important tests in diagnosing allergies.

Chapter 5

Diagnosing Allergies

The diagnosis of an allergy is important. For many people with allergies, symptoms are annoying or uncomfortable. Allergies can be serious or dangerous for people with severe allergic reactions. The correct diagnosis can lead to appropriate treatment and relief for these people.

Farms and fields contain lots of dust, mold, and pollen.

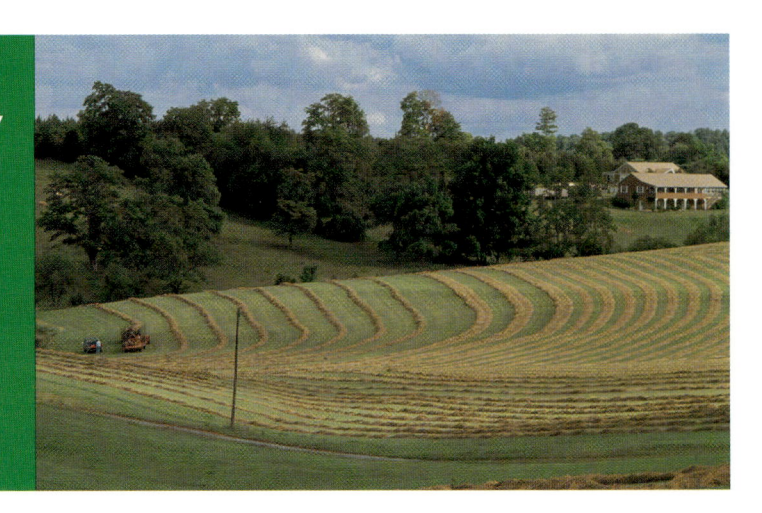

Rosa, Age 17

Rosa lived in a big city all her life. When her family moved to a small farm town, Rosa sneezed a lot in the spring. She had a stuffy and itchy nose. Her eyes were red and sore. She could go through a box of tissues in a couple of days from all her sneezing.

Rosa's parents worried about her. Also, they needed Rosa's help with the yard work, but she felt the worst when she was outside. Her parents thought Rosa might have allergies. They wanted her to see a doctor.

Allergy Symptoms

Diagnosing allergies can be difficult at times. Symptoms sometimes are similar to those of other common diseases. For example, hay fever symptoms mimic cold symptoms. But there are differences. Doctors can use these differences in symptoms to diagnose allergies correctly.

> **Fast Fact**
>
> The Greek doctor Hippocrates noted the first food allergy in the fourth century B.C. He wrote that milk caused an upset stomach and hives in some people.

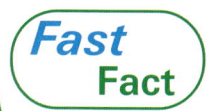

Allergy symptoms vary from person to person. Different allergies affect different body areas. Symptoms may appear suddenly, or they may be constant. The chart shows some physical symptoms of allergies.

Allergy Symptoms

Mild to moderate symptoms	
Hives or a red, itchy rash	Upset stomach
Sneezing, stuffy nose	Burning or itchy mouth and lips
Puffy face	
Red, watery eyes	

Severe symptoms	
Hives all over the body	Fainting
Red face	Falling blood pressure
Swollen tongue	Voice changes, difficulty speaking
Trouble swallowing	
Rapid pulse	Wheezing or shortness of breath

Diagnosing Allergies

A doctor can tell you if you have allergies. You'll probably have a physical exam.

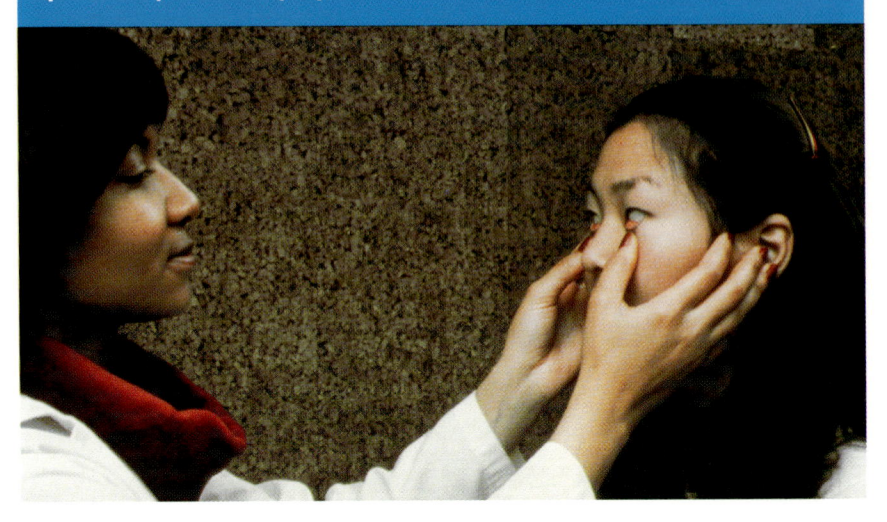

There are other signs of allergies. People with an allergy may be irritable because of discomfort. They may dislike outdoor activities if they react to pollen or mold. They may avoid going places where they might have allergic reactions.

Steps in Diagnosis

Diagnosing allergies involves several steps. Doctors take the person's medical history. They want to know about the person's health in the past. If you are being diagnosed, doctors will ask if your parents have allergies. They also will ask about your lifestyle, diet, and home life.

Rosa's Exam

Rosa went to her family doctor. Rosa's doctor thought she might have several allergies. To be sure, he sent Rosa to an allergist. This is a doctor who specializes in diagnosing and treating allergies.

The allergist first took Rosa's medical history. She wanted to know if anyone in Rosa's family had allergies and when those started. Then she asked these questions about Rosa's symptoms:

Do your symptoms get worse during certain months?

Do you have pets? If yes, do your symptoms get better when you're away from home? Do your symptoms return or get worse when you get home?

Do your eyes or skin itch and redden after playing with your pet? If your pet licks you, do you get any symptoms?

Do you sneeze when the carpets are vacuumed?

Do you develop symptoms when you go into a damp basement?

Do your symptoms start after you eat certain foods?

Next came a physical examination. The allergist listened to Rosa's breathing. She checked Rosa's breathing muscles. She also examined Rosa's eyes, ears, nose, and throat for signs of infection.

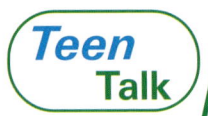

> **Teen Talk**
>
> "My dad thought I had allergies. He wanted me to see a doctor. This doctor said I should be tested for 200 to 300 allergens. My dad thought that sounded strange. He checked with other doctors who said that was too many allergens to test for."
> —Larry, age 14

Then the allergist did a skin test. Skin tests are most important in determining which allergens cause a reaction. The allergist used a small, plastic device to prick Rosa's skin with a tiny amount of 10 allergens. The skin pricks took about 2 minutes. The allergist had Rosa wait 15 minutes to see if a reaction appeared. Rosa had a raised red spot on some of her skin tests. The spots looked like mosquito bites. The skin test area also itched and turned a little red.

The allergist gave Rosa some lotion to help stop the itching. She told Rosa that the redness would fade within an hour.

Other Tests

Allergists may use other tests such as the following to confirm allergies:

> Injection tests are best for drug and insect allergies. A tiny amount of allergen is injected by needle just below the skin.
>
> Patch tests can identify skin allergies. Small patches of material are covered with the allergen. Then the patches are put on the back or arm and left for 48 hours.

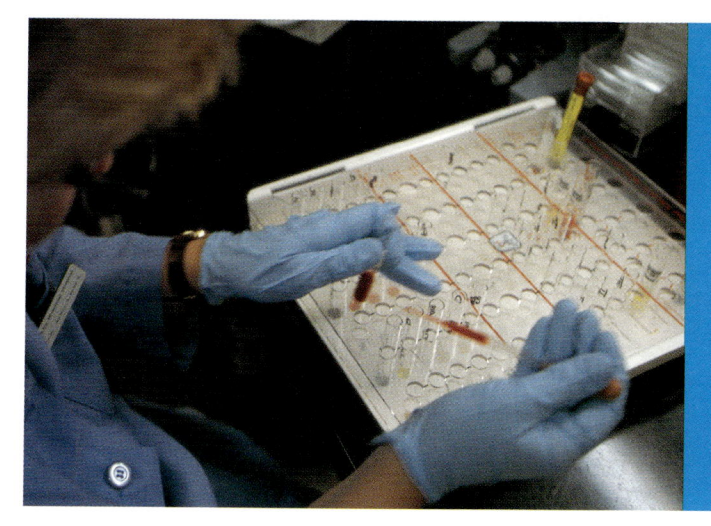

Blood tests are one way to check for allergies. The results may take longer than other tests to receive.

Food tests are extremely sensitive. People stop eating one or more foods that may cause an allergic reaction. If symptoms disappear, the person starts to eat each food separately to see if symptoms return.

Blood tests are used if the person could have a severe allergic reaction to an allergen. The results take a week or more.

Rosa's Diagnosis

The allergist confirmed that Rosa had allergies. She was allergic to tree and grass pollens and to mold. Rosa's allergies were worst in the spring and fall. Rosa's parents weren't surprised. They both had hay fever every spring.

Rosa will be fine. She's receiving treatment. She can still help with the yard work. Her parents will help Rosa manage her allergies.

Points to Consider

How would you feel if a doctor said you had allergies?

How would you convince someone you thought had an allergy to see a doctor?

How do you react when you have to get a shot?

Chapter Overview

Allergies can be controlled or even cured. With proper treatment, people with allergies can be as active as they like.

Avoiding allergy triggers is the most basic way to control allergies.

Allergy medications are helpful in controlling allergies. A variety of drugs are available. Over-the-counter allergy drugs work for some people. Others need prescription drugs.

Some people find relief from allergy symptoms through a series of allergy shots. This treatment can take one to two years, or even longer. Shots work only for certain allergies.

Chapter 6

Controlling Allergies

Proper treatment can control or even cure allergies. Control means that an allergy doesn't interfere with a healthy, normal life. People with allergies can achieve control by following their treatment program. Treatment plans vary from person to person and depend on the symptoms and severity of the allergy.

Scientists are working to better understand why the immune system gets mixed up. This helps them develop better ways to diagnose, treat, and prevent allergies. Scientists study how the immune system works in allergic reactions. They can use this information to look for new ways to stop allergic reactions from occurring. They also hope to find better allergy treatments and anti-allergy vaccines.

Guinea pigs are sometimes found in school classrooms. Work with school staff members to remove allergy triggers like this.

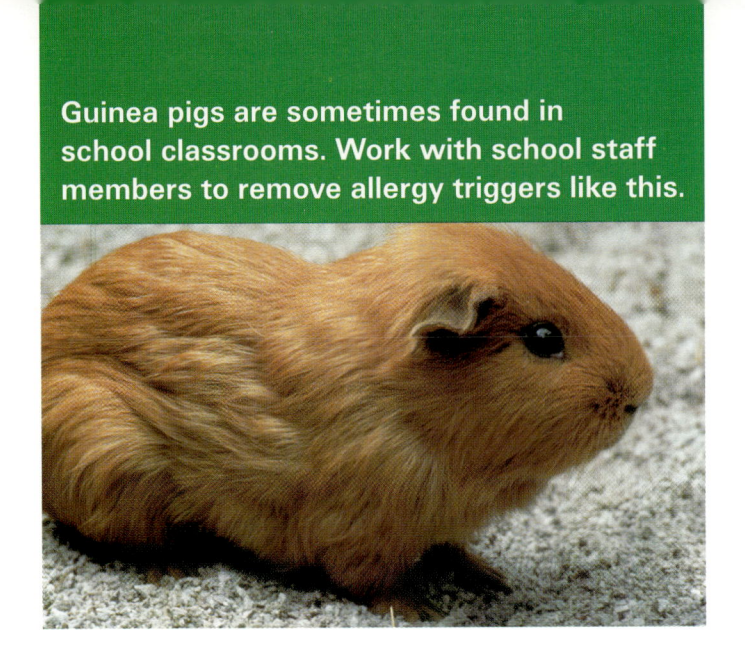

Avoiding Allergy Triggers

The most obvious way to control an allergy is to figure out the cause. Then, if possible, the person can avoid it or remove it from their surroundings. By avoiding triggers, people with allergies may have fewer or no allergic reactions. Their reactions may be less severe. People with allergies might discover their triggers through trial and error. Allergy testing also can reveal the source.

Children and teens with allergies may encounter allergy triggers at school. Some common triggers at school include dust, dust mites, and cockroaches. Science classes may be home to rats, guinea pigs, and other furry animals. If these are triggers, ask school staff members to help in removing them or helping students avoid them.

Medications

Medications can play an important part in controlling allergies. There are several classes of medications. The main class is antihistamines. These drugs block the effect of histamines. They work fast during an allergy attack to stop itching, sneezing, and a runny nose. Some earlier antihistamines can make the user feel sleepy or tired. Newer antihistamines don't have this side effect.

Fast Fact

For hay fever relief, people spend $2.4 million on drugs and $1.1 billion in medical bills each year.

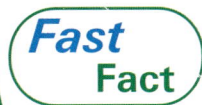

A second class of medications is anti-inflammatories, which reduce swelling in the air tubes. This makes the tubes less sensitive to triggers and eases breathing.

Decongestants are a third class of allergy drugs. They reduce nasal congestion or stuffiness. They're sold without a prescription, or doctor's order. Decongestants don't stop runny noses, sneezing, or itching.

Allergy drugs are delivered in different ways. One way is through nasal sprays. It's best to use a nasal spray before the start of allergy season and continue until the season has ended. Pills and injections are other delivery methods.

People with mild allergies may find that over-the-counter allergy drugs relieve their symptoms. These drugs contain a mixture of ingredients. People with moderate to severe allergies often need prescription drugs. A doctor prescribes a medicine and dosage that fit the person. People with allergies always should take medicines exactly as prescribed. They should tell their doctor if the medicine isn't working.

Many schools have specific procedures students must follow to carry or use medicines.

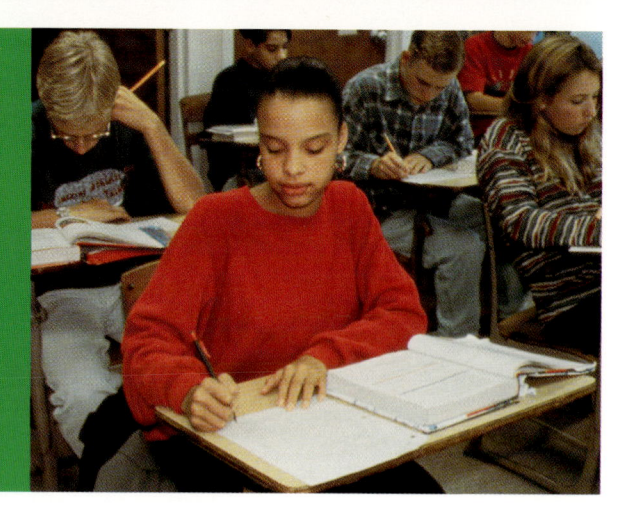

Alex, Age 13

Alex is allergic to grass and weed pollen. "I'd feel lousy during the spring and summer. Instead of having fun with my friends, I'd be home with a box of tissues. Finally, Dad took me to a doctor, who prescribed a nasal spray. She showed me how to do two sprays in each nostril. She said to use it once a day, and things would improve after five days. It worked! I felt better in five days. After two weeks, my symptoms were gone. Now I use the spray during the allergy season and never have a problem."

Taking Allergy Medications

Allergy medications can be taken in a variety of ways. Some are swallowed or injected with a needle. Others are sprayed or dropped into the nose.

Children and teens with allergies may need to take medication during the school day. Parents or guardians should tell school staff members the child's medication plan. They need to know if the child needs help taking the medication. Some schools don't allow students to carry medication with them. These schools say that all medications must be kept in the nurse's office. Other schools allow students to carry medicine but specify where students can take it. For example, a student may step into the hall to use a nasal spray.

Myth: It may take months or even years before allergy shots start to work.

Fact: Most people start to feel better quickly after starting a series of allergy shots.

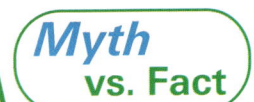

Myth vs. Fact

Allergy Shots

Some people find relief from their allergy symptoms after they get a series of allergy shots. The shots increase a person's tolerance to an allergen. This process usually takes one to two years but can take as long as five years. If the treatment works, allergic symptoms decrease or disappear.

The shots may be given once a week. Over time, the dose increases slightly. After 15 to 30 weeks, shots are needed only every four to six weeks or so. Children younger than age 5 can't get allergy shots.

Allergy shots work best if the exact allergens are known. Pollen allergies often are treated successfully through shots. Allergies to dust mites, pets, molds, and stings from hornets, wasps, and bees also can be treated successfully. Allergy shots aren't used for eczema, food allergies, or drug allergies.

Did You Know?

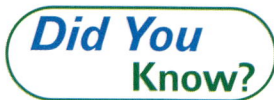

Qualified experts know a lot about what causes allergies.

"My allergies got worse each year. When I was 10, my doctor determined I had pollen and mold allergies. My parents and I talked with my doctor and decided to try allergy shots. The doctor said the shots might not work. I could have an allergic reaction to them. And they would take time. I had to sit in the doctor's office about 20 minutes after getting a shot. That was to make sure I didn't have a bad reaction.

Sasha, Age 12

"At first, I got a shot once a week in my upper arm. The nurse used a tiny needle. The spot itched and turned a little red but didn't hurt much. Even the itching and redness stopped after awhile. After six months, my symptoms weren't so bad. Then the doctor said I only needed to come in once a month for a shot.

"I've had two years of shots and don't have any symptoms. I go outside whenever I want. My doctor says I have to get shots for another year, just to be sure."

At a Glance

Deaths from severe allergy attacks are rare. About 500 people in the United States and 50 people in Canada die from anaphylaxis each year. Anaphylaxis is a severe allergy attack.

Points to Consider

What in your school might trigger an allergy?

What is your school's policy about carrying prescription drugs? If you don't know, how could you find out?

Why do you think schools might not allow students to carry prescription drugs?

Why might it be hard for a teen to stick to an allergy shot treatment program?

Chapter Overview

People with allergies should be prepared for anaphylaxis. They should know their allergy warning signals and discuss an emergency action plan with their doctor. They need a supply of medication on hand.

People with severe allergies should inform family, friends, teachers, and coworkers about their condition. These people may need to assist the person with allergies during anaphylaxis.

Smoking can make an allergy reaction worse. It also can make recovery from a severe attack more difficult.

Chapter 7

Handling an Allergy Attack

Some people have sudden, severe allergy attacks called anaphylaxis. There may be no warning ahead of time that this could happen. Anaphylaxis could occur even with proper treatment. Many people try to avoid their trigger, but they could come into contact with it without warning.

Such severe attacks could result in death. Anaphylaxis can be frightening not only for the person having the attack but also for anybody watching. Knowing what to do can help ease people's fears and even save lives.

Early Warning Signals

Certain signals might occur at the start of a severe allergy attack. They warn the person that worse symptoms are coming. The signals can be seen and felt. The next page shows examples of signals.

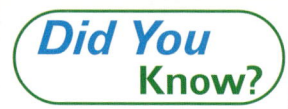

> **Did You Know?** Doctors can't predict with certainty if an allergy can cause someone to be at high risk for a severe reaction.

- Severe itching
- Hives
- Upset stomach
- Headache
- Skin that turns red and warm
- Tongue or throat that swells

Every person with an allergy has an individual pattern of signals. People can learn to identify their signals. They should discuss with their doctor what to do when their early warning signals occur. Adult caregivers need to be alert to warning signals in children with allergies. That way, they can provide immediate help.

Late Warning Signals

Certain signals may appear as anaphylaxis becomes worse. They warn that the person could collapse and possibly die. The signals affect all body systems. Some examples of late signals include:

- Drop in blood pressure
- Weak pulse
- Difficulty swallowing
- Wheezing and difficulty breathing
- Stomach pain or cramps
- Nausea or vomiting
- Muscle weakness
- Fainting

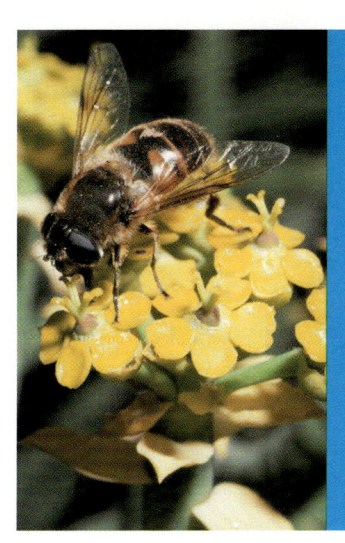

Anaphylaxis is a life-threatening allergic reaction. Bee stings may cause anaphylaxis.

Janna, Age 16

Janna was 4 years old the first time a bee stung her. A small red bump appeared where she was stung. It hurt for a day and then went away. When Janna was 12, another bee stung her. Her mom took the stinger out and wiped her arm with rubbing alcohol. This time, Janna's reaction was different. After 15 minutes, Janna felt sick and had a headache. Then hives appeared all over her body, and she had trouble breathing. Her mom called 9-1-1.

A bee sting caused anaphylaxis in Janna. She needed emergency medical treatment. People having a severe allergy attack may be hospitalized. They may need oxygen to help protect the heart and brain. They may need fluids to raise blood pressure and pull them out of shock. They also may need medicine to reduce the swelling of air passages and to counter hives.

Prepare for an Emergency

Liz, Age 15

"I'm allergic to peanuts and always avoid them. When I was 12, a tiny bit of peanut got into my food. I fainted and had to go to the emergency room. I was okay, but the doctor told me to carry a shot of epinephrine. He said it could save my life someday."

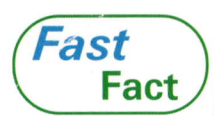

Fast Fact: Allergens most likely to trigger anaphylaxis are drugs, insect stings, and some foods.

People like Liz with a severe allergic reaction may not have time to get to the emergency room. Their throat can close up, and they could stop breathing. These people always should carry a dose of epinephrine, a substance that helps the body reverse severe allergic reactions. Epinephrine also is called adrenaline.

One device with epinephrine is about the size and shape of a pen. To use the device, a person pulls off the safety cap and jabs the pen against the thigh. A needle springs out and releases a dose of epinephrine. Some people with severe allergic reactions carry an injection kit. Using either system takes just a few seconds. Getting a shot is the fastest way to get a medicine into a person. A doctor needs to prescribe epinephrine. A doctor also will have a training pen with no needle to practice the injection.

Emergency epinephrine should be used at the first sign of a reaction and could save a person's life. It provides about 15 minutes of relief. Such an emergency shot isn't a substitute for medical help. A person who has had anaphylaxis still needs to go to an emergency room right away.

Anaphylaxis in School

Teens and children with severe allergy reactions may have an attack at school. Parents need to prepare school personnel to deal with an attack. The principal, school nurse, and teachers should have a written rescue plan. Such a plan contains this information:

- Symptoms of a student's allergy attacks
- Steps to take during an attack
- When to seek emergency care
- Person or persons to contact in an emergency
- Emergency allergy medications and how to give them

Cigarette smoke may trigger an allergic reaction or worsen side effects of allergy medicines.

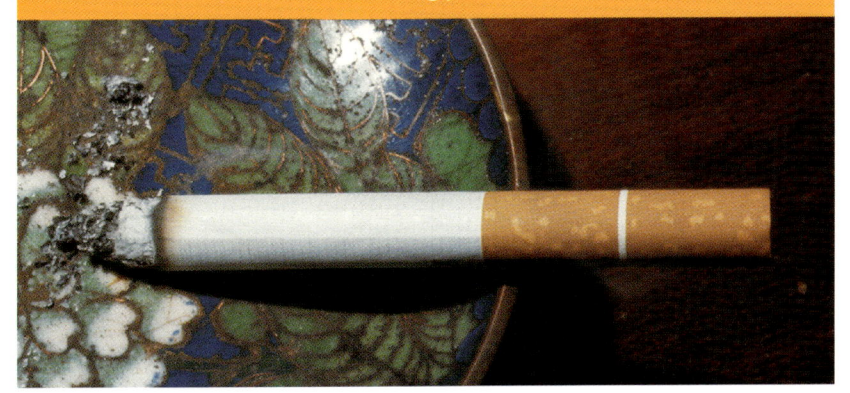

Tobacco

Smoking can be dangerous for anyone. It's especially dangerous for people with allergies. It can contain allergy triggers and might cause an attack. Smoking can make asthma worse, and secondhand smoke can cause allergies in infants.

Points to Consider

Why might children and teens with severe allergies have a high number of emergency room visits?

Whom should teens with moderate to severe allergies tell about their condition?

What could you do to help a person during anaphylaxis?

Why should people with allergies avoid tobacco and other drugs?

Glossary

allergen (AL-ur-juhn)—something that causes an allergic reaction

allergic reaction (uh-LUR-jik ree-AK-shuhn)—the body's rejection of and reaction to a substance in or touching the body

allergist (AL-ur-jist)—a doctor who specializes in diagnosing and treating allergies

anaphylaxis (an-uh-fuh-LAK-suhss)—a severe, sudden allergy attack

antibody (AN-ti-bod-ee)—a substance that fights off harmful invaders in the body; special white blood cells in the immune system produce antibodies.

chronic (KRON-ik)—continuing for a long time

dietitian (dye-uh-TISH-uhn)—a nutrition expert who can teach people with allergies which foods to avoid

eczema (EK-suh-muh)—a chronic skin allergy that causes itchy skin rashes

epinephrine (ep-uh-NEF-ruhn)—a substance that helps the body cope with a severe allergic reaction; epinephrine also is called adrenaline.

histamine (HISS-tuh-meen)—a chemical released by the immune system during an allergic reaction

hives (HIVEZ)—red, itchy bumps on the skin that an allergy may cause

immune system (i-MYOON SISS-tuhm)—the system that protects the body from illness and disease; it produces cells that attack viruses and bacteria.

inflame (in-FLAME)—to cause redness, swelling, heat, and pain

intolerance (in-TOL-ur-uhnss)—the body's negative reaction to a food, drug, or other substance

pathogen (PATH-uh-juhn)—disease-causing agent such as bacteria or a virus

For More Information

Edelson, Edward. *Allergies*. Broomall, PA: Chelsea House, 1999.

Moragne, Wendy. *Allergies*. Brookfield, CT: Millbrook, 1999.

Peacock, Judith. *Asthma*. Mankato, MN: Capstone, 2000.

Silverstein, Alvin, Virginia Silverstein, and Laura Silverstein Nunn. *Allergies*. New York: Franklin Watts, 1999.

Useful Addresses and Internet Sites

Allergy and Asthma Network
2751 Prosperity Avenue, Suite 150
Fairfax, VA 22031-4397
1-800-878-4403
www.aanma.org

American Academy of Allergy, Asthma, and Immunology
611 East Wells Street
Milwaukee, WI 53202
www.aaaai.org

American College of Allergy, Asthma, and Immunology
85 West Algonquin Road, Suite 550
Arlington Heights, IL 60005
http://allergy.mcg.edu

Asthma and Allergy Foundation of America
1233 20th Street Northwest, Suite 402
Washington, DC 20036
1-800-7-ASTHMA (1-800-727-8462)
www.aafa.org

Canadian Lung Association
3 Raymond Street, Suite 300
Ottawa, ON K1R 1A3
CANADA
www.lung.ca

Food Allergy Network
10400 Eaton Place, Suite 107
Fairfax, VA 22030-2208
1-800-929-4040
www.foodallergy.org
www.foodallergy.org/canadaalerts.html
(Food alerts in Canada)

National Institute of Allergy and Infectious Diseases (NIAID)
Office of Communications and Public Liaison
Building 31, Room 7A-50
31 Center Drive MSC 2520
Bethesda, MD 20892-2520
www.niaid.nih.gov

Allergy ABCs
http://allergyabcs.com/allergies.htm
Information for young people about allergies

Mayo Clinic: Allergy and Asthma Center
www.mayohealth.org/mayo/common/htm/allergy.htm
Articles and links about allergies

About.Com Health for Teens: Allergies and Asthma
http://teenhealth.about.com/teens/teenhealth/msub03.htm
Articles for teens about allergies

Index

air conditioners, 19, 20, 32, 34
allergies. *See also* animal allergies; drug allergies; food allergies; plant allergies; skin allergies
    avoiding, 16, 19, 20, 21, 26, 28, 36, 48, 55
    controlling, 47–53
    cures, 47
    defined, 5–11
    diagnosing, 39–45
    seasonal, 6, 13–21
    symptoms of, 7–8, 11, 24, 25, 27, 40–43, 56
    triggers of, 5, 8–11, 13–21, 48
    types of, 14–15, 23, 31–37
    who get them?, 6, 10–11
allergists, 29, 42–45
allergy attacks, 35, 53, 55–59
anaphylaxis, 53, 55–59
    early warning signals of, 55, 56
    late warning signals of, 56–57
animal allergies, 5, 8, 9, 18, 33–35, 48. *See also* cockroaches; pets
antibodies, 7, 26
antihistamines, 48
anti-inflammatories, 49
asthma, 6, 10, 59

bacteria, 7, 24, 25
blisters, 24
blood tests, 45
breathing, 6, 8, 10, 15, 19, 27, 41, 43, 49, 56, 57. *See also* asthma; wheezing

cats, 33, 34
cleaning, 20, 21, 26, 29, 32, 34, 35, 43
cockroaches, 31, 35, 48

death, 6, 27, 36, 53, 55, 56
decongestants, 49
dehumidifiers, 20
dietitians, 29
dogs, 33–34
drug allergies, 9, 31, 36–37, 44, 51
dust, 10, 19, 31–33, 34, 35, 40, 48
dust mites, 9, 31–33, 48, 51

eczema, 25, 51
eggs, 27
emergencies, 57
epinephrine, 57, 58
eyes, 5, 7, 8, 10, 14, 19, 24, 33, 40, 41, 43

fainting, 27, 41, 56
fish, 27
food allergies, 5, 8, 9, 10, 23, 31, 43, 51
    coping with, 28–29
    defined, 26–27
    symptoms of, 27
    who gets them?, 27
food labels, 28, 29
food tests, 45

grass, 16–17, 45, 50

hair dye, 25
hay fever, 9, 13–21, 45
    coping with triggers, 19–21
    defined, 14–15
    and mold triggers, 18–19
    and pollen triggers, 15–17
    symptoms, 10, 14–15, 40
    who gets it?, 15
headaches, 14, 15, 56, 57
histamine, 7, 14, 26, 48

Index continued

hives, 8, 41, 56, 57
humidity, 32

immune system, 7, 11, 26, 34, 36, 47
infections, 24, 25, 43
injections, 9, 47, 49, 50, 51–52, 57, 58
injection tests, 44
insects, 9, 19, 32, 44, 51, 57
itching, 5, 8, 10, 14, 24, 25, 40, 41, 43, 44, 48–49, 52, 56

medications, 48–50, 57, 58
metals, 25
milk, 10, 27, 29, 41
mold, 9, 10, 13, 14, 40, 45, 51–52
    reducing levels of, 20–21
    triggers for hay fever, 18–19, 21, 40, 42
myths, 9, 14, 34, 51

nasal sprays, 49, 50
nose, runny, 7, 8, 14, 48–49
nuts, 27

patch tests, 44
peanuts, 27, 57
penicillin, 36
pets, 31, 33–34, 43, 51
pills, 49, 50
plant allergies, 5, 8, 25. *See also* hay fever
pollen, 9, 10, 13, 14, 31, 40, 45, 50, 51–52
    reducing indoor, 20
    triggers for hay fever, 15–17, 19, 21, 42

rashes, 8, 24, 25, 26, 37, 41

school, 48, 50, 58
scratching, 5, 26
seasonal allergies, 6, 52. *See also* hay fever
shellfish, 5, 7, 27
skin allergies, 23, 24, 56
    allergic eczema, 25
    coping with, 26
    defined, 24–25
skin tests, 44
smoking, 19, 59
sneezing, 8, 10, 14, 21, 33, 40, 41, 43, 48–49
stomachaches, 8, 27, 41, 56, 57
swelling, 5, 14, 24, 27, 41, 49, 56, 57

testing, 44–45, 48
throat, sore, 8, 14, 15
tobacco, 59
training pen, 58
treatment plans, 47–52
trees, 14, 16–17, 45

vaccines. *See* injections

weeds, 9, 14, 16–17, 50
wheezing, 8, 10, 41, 56. *See also* breathing

yards, 18–19, 20, 21, 40, 45
year-round allergies, 6